It's easy to get lost in the cancer world

Let NCCN Guidelines for Patients® be your guide

- ✓ Step-by-step guides to the cancer care options likely to have the best results
- ✓ Based on treatment guidelines used by health care providers worldwide
- ✓ Designed to help you discuss cancer treatment with your doctors

National Comprehensive Cancer Network®

NCCN Guidelines for Patients® are developed by the National Comprehensive Cancer Network® (NCCN®)

NCCN®

- An alliance of 28 leading cancer centers across the United States devoted to patient care, research, and education

Cancer centers that are part of NCCN:
NCCN.org/cancercenters

NCCN Clinical Practice Guidelines in Oncology (NCCN Guidelines®)

- Developed by doctors from NCCN cancer centers using the latest research and years of experience
- For providers of cancer care all over the world
- Expert recommendations for cancer screening, diagnosis, and treatment

Free online at
NCCN.org/guidelines

NCCN Guidelines for Patients®

- Present information from the NCCN Guidelines in an easy-to-learn format
- For people with cancer and those who support them
- Explain the cancer care options likely to have the best results

NCCN Quick Guide™ Sheets

- Key points from the NCCN Guidelines for Patients

Free online at
NCCN.org/patientguidelines

NATIONAL COMPREHENSIVE CANCER NETWORK FOUNDATION
Guiding Treatment. Changing Lives.

and supported by funding from NCCN Foundation®

These guidelines are based on the NCCN Clinical Practice Guidelines in Oncology (NCCN Guidelines®) for Lung Cancer Screening (Version 1.2020, May 14, 2019).

NCCN Foundation® seeks to support the millions of patients and their families affected by a cancer diagnosis by funding and distributing NCCN Guidelines for Patients®. NCCN Foundation is also committed to advancing cancer treatment by funding the nation's promising doctors at the center of innovation in cancer research. For more details and the full library of patient and caregiver resources, visit NCCN.org/patients. We rely solely on donations to fund the NCCN Guidelines for Patients. To donate, visit NCCNFoundation.org/Donate.

National Comprehensive Cancer Network® (NCCN®) and NCCN Foundation®
3025 Chemical Road, Suite 100 | Plymouth Meeting, PA 19462 | 215.690.0300

Endorsed by

American Lung Association
The American Lung Association strongly supports efforts to help ensure all patients facing lung cancer get the highest standard of treatment and care. Helping patients understand treatment guidelines is one important step in empowering them to get the care they want and need. That is why we are pleased to endorse NCCN'S efforts to provide accessible treatment guidelines and information to patients through the NCCN Guidelines for Patients. Lung.org

Bonnie J. Addario Lung Cancer Foundation
The Bonnie J. Addario Lung Cancer Foundation is proud to endorse these NCCN Guidelines for Patients. We believe that educated and empowered patients live longer. This book should be in the hands of every patient diagnosed with lung cancer. lungcancerfoundation.org

Caring Ambassadors
The Caring Ambassador Lung Cancer Program is pleased to endorse these NCCN Guidelines for Patients: Non-Small Cell Lung Cancer. Patients and their loved ones need reliable resources to achieve the best possible outcomes for their disease. lungcancercap.org

Dusty Joy Foundation (LiveLung)
With patients' best interest at heart, NCCN defines the standard of care for patients and physicians through proven scientific methods and expectations for new discoveries leading to improved patient outcomes. As a lung cancer advocacy nonprofit, our organization wholeheartedly supports the NCCN Guidelines for Patients. LiveLung.org

Free ME from Lung Cancer
As a lung cancer survivor and President and CEO of Free ME from Lung Cancer, I am pleased to endorse this vitally important resource so that lung cancer patients can have the information needed to make informed decisions about their treatment. freeMEfromLungCancer.org

Lung Cancer Action Network (LungCAN)
The NCCN provides the most current standards for patient care in an easy-to-understand and highly accessible format. As a collaborative association of approximately 25 U.S.-based nonprofits dedicated to lung cancer, the Lung Cancer Action Network (LungCAN) is proud to endorse NCCN Guidelines for Lung Cancer Patients. LungCAN.org

Lung Cancer Alliance
Lung Cancer Alliance is proud to collaborate with the National Comprehensive Cancer Network to endorse these NCCN Guidelines for Patients®: Non-Small Cell Lung Cancer. lungcanceralliance.org

Lung Cancer Circle of Hope
Lung Cancer Circle of Hope (LCCH) emphatically endorses the NCCN Guidelines for Patients. Knowledge is power and with this comprehensive resource, patients and their families can proactively work with a qualified physician to make informed decisions in the battle to conquer cancer. lungcancercircleofhope.org

Lung Cancer Initiative of North Carolina
As an organization specializing in connecting patients, survivors and loved ones with the medical research community, the Lung Cancer Initiative of NC fully supports these NCCN Guidelines for Patients. These guidelines set the standard for patient education and access to care. lungcancerinitiativenc.org

Lung Cancer Research Foundation
As a non-profit organization focused on supporting lung cancer research, the Lung Cancer Research Foundation is proud to endorse the NCCN Guidelines for Patients. These guidelines play an important role in providing lung cancer patients with up to date information and empowering them to make informed decisions about their care. lcrf.org

LUNGevity
LUNGevity Foundation supports the NCCN Guidelines for Patients as an excellent resource, as we strongly believe in providing education for all those affected by the disease. LUNGevity.org

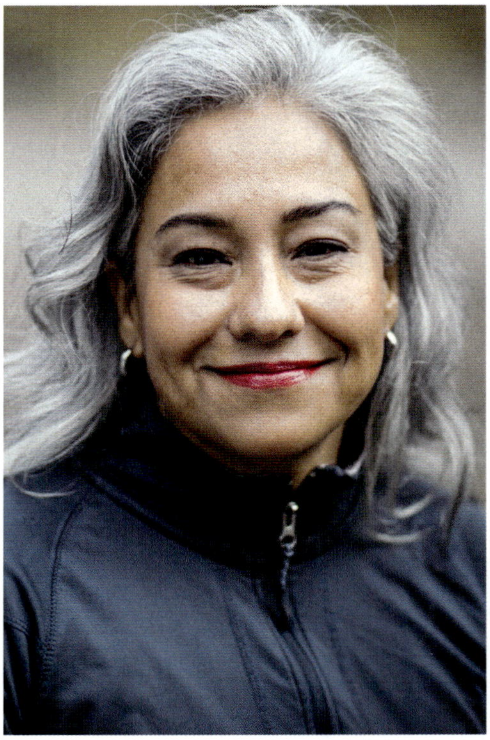
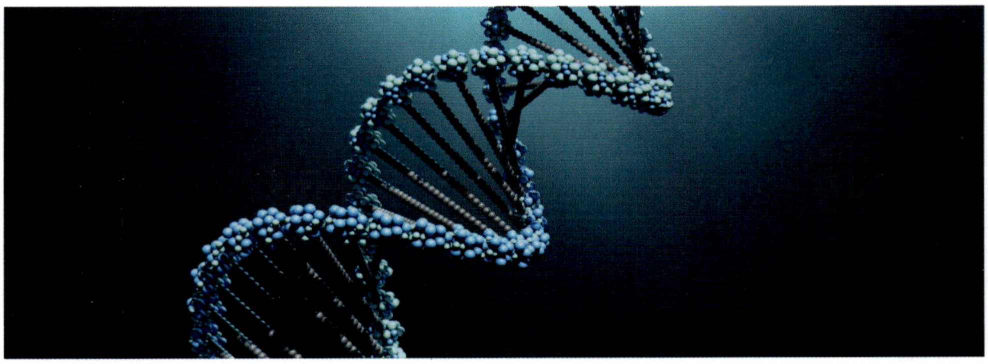
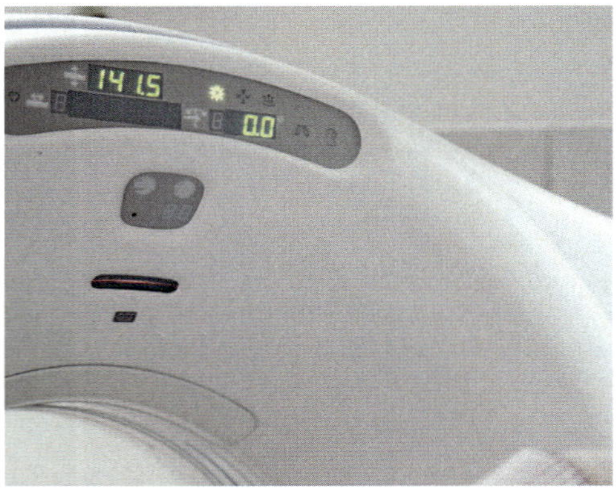
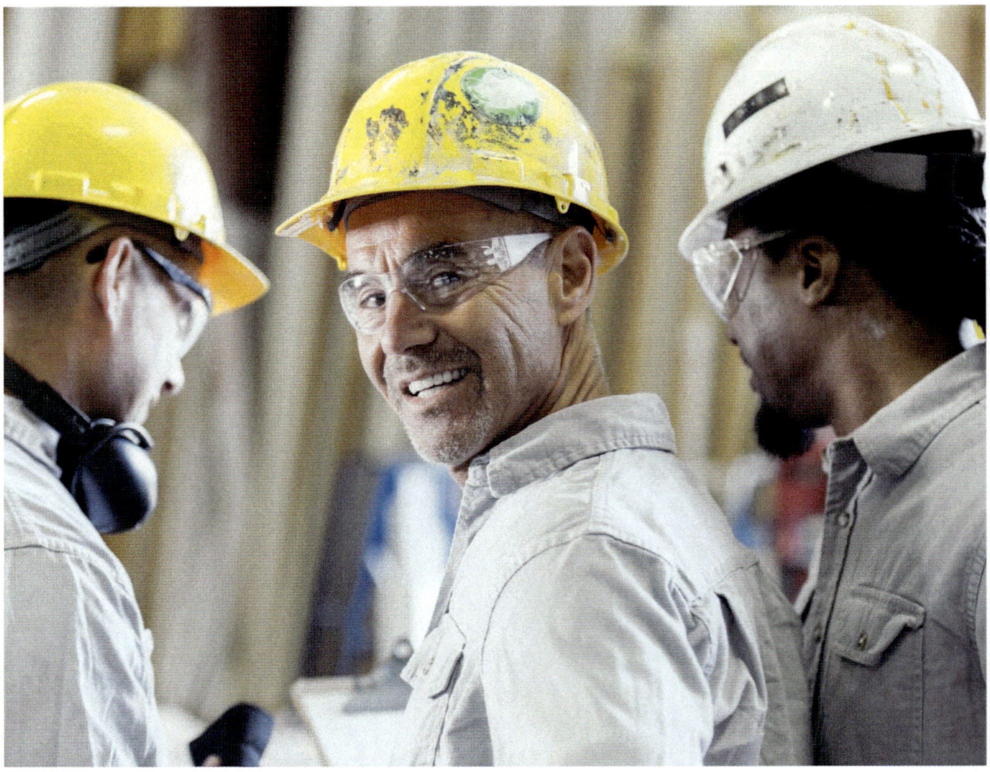
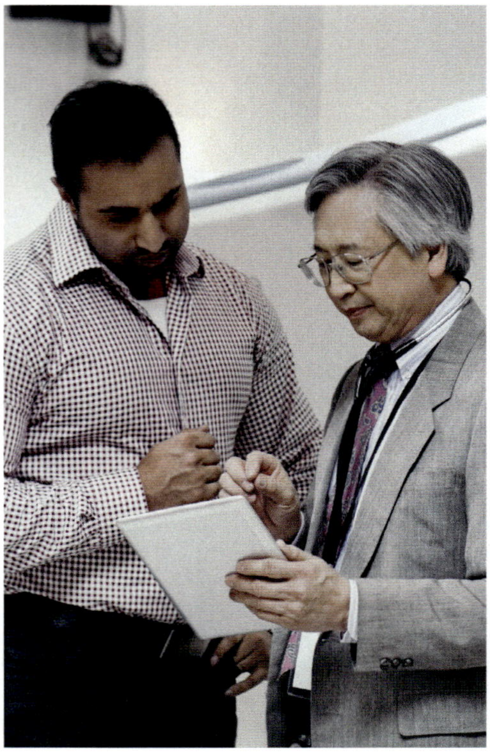
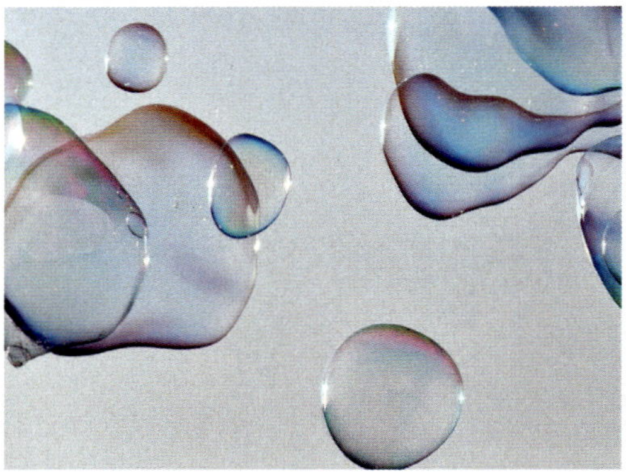
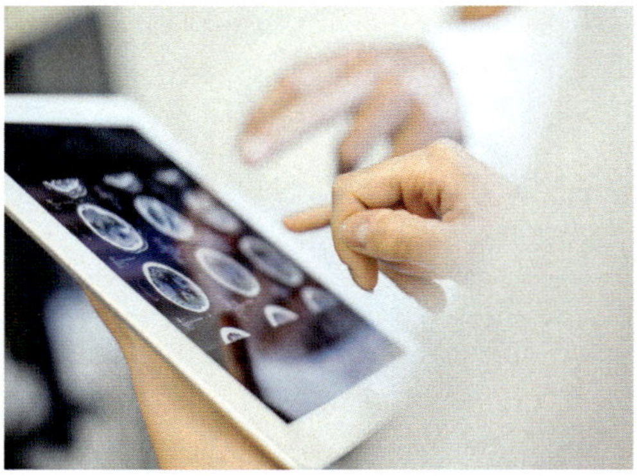
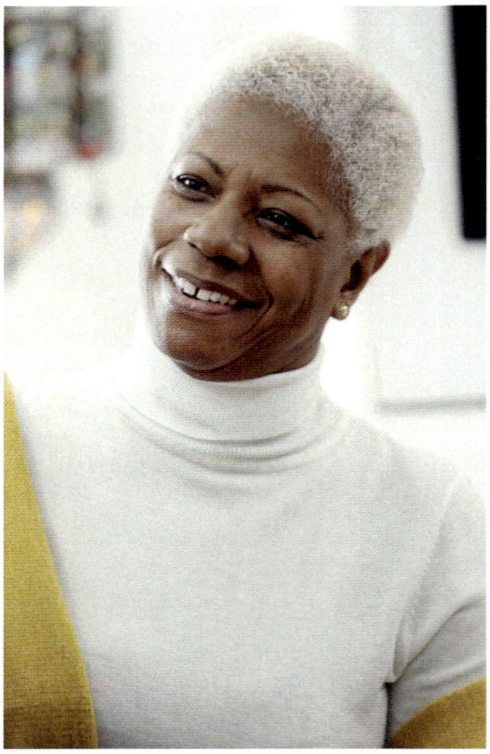

Contents

1
Why get screened?

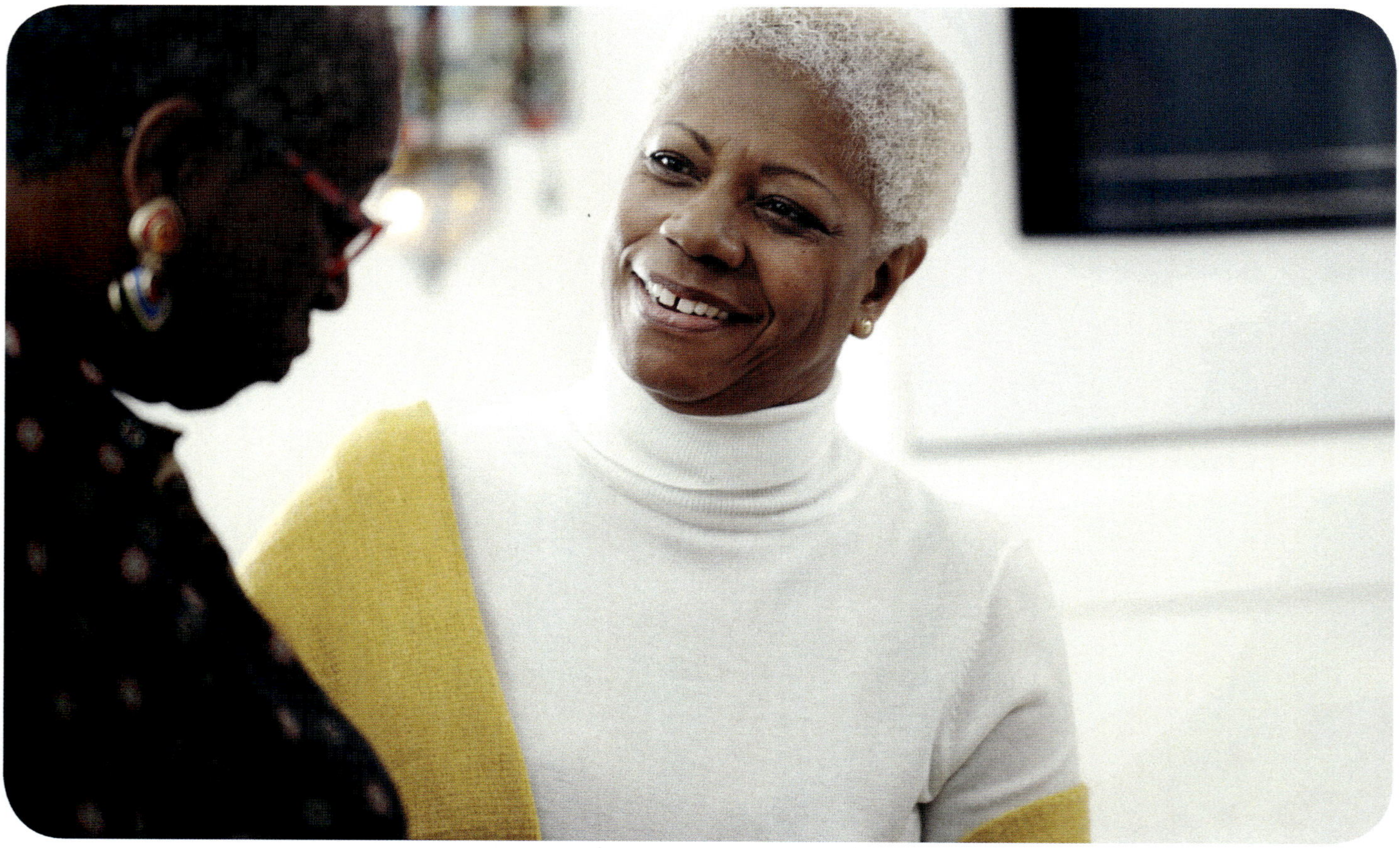

The lungs

The lungs are a pair of organs in the chest that are vital to life. The lungs move important gases in and out of the blood. You breathe in oxygen and exhale carbon dioxide (a gas made by cells) from the body.

The lungs have sections called lobes. The left lung has 2 lobes and the right lung has 3 lobes. A thin layer of tissue (membrane) surrounds the lungs called the pleural membrane. This membrane protects the lungs.

Two large breathing tubes, called bronchi, connect the windpipe (trachea) to the lungs. There is one tube, called a bronchus, for each lung. Inside the lungs are small tubes (bronchioles) and small air sacs (alveoli). **See Figure 1**.

2.5 out of 10 cancer deaths are from lung cancer

Figure 1
The lungs

The lungs have sections called lobes. The left lung has 2 lobes and the right lung has 3 lobes.

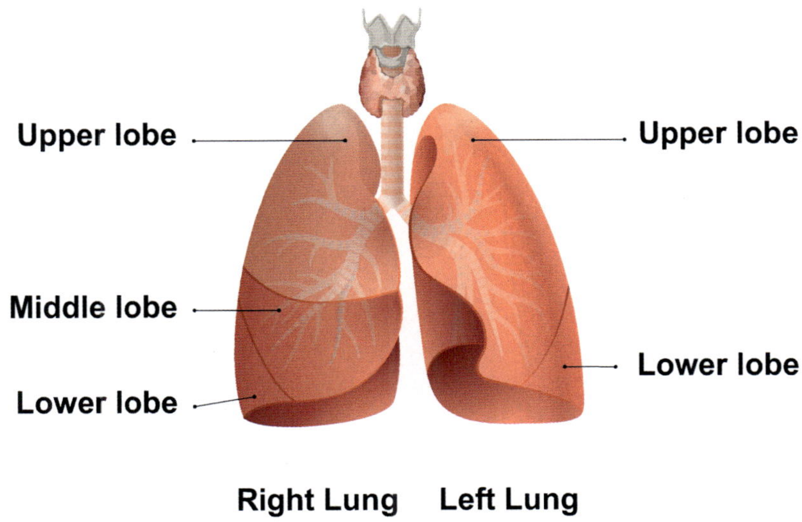

Detect lung cancer early

Lung cancer is a disease that starts in the cells that make up the lungs. Normal cells make new cells when needed, die when old or damaged, and stay in place. Cancer cells don't do this. They grow out of control and invade other tissue. Without treatment, cancer cells can form a tumor (abnormal mass of cells) and spread to other organs in the body.

Lung cancer is the leading cause of cancer deaths in the United States and the world. **See Figures 2 and 3**. The goal of lung cancer screening is to catch lung cancer early, at a stage before there are any symptoms. This is when treatment will be most successful. Once you have symptoms like a cough that won't go away, it is usually too late to cure lung cancer. Early detection of lung cancer helps prevent death. Your doctor will look at your risk factors for lung cancer before recommending screening. Together, you will make an informed decision on whether screening is an appropriate option for you.

Figure 2
Lung cancer in the United States

1 out of 14 people develop lung cancer

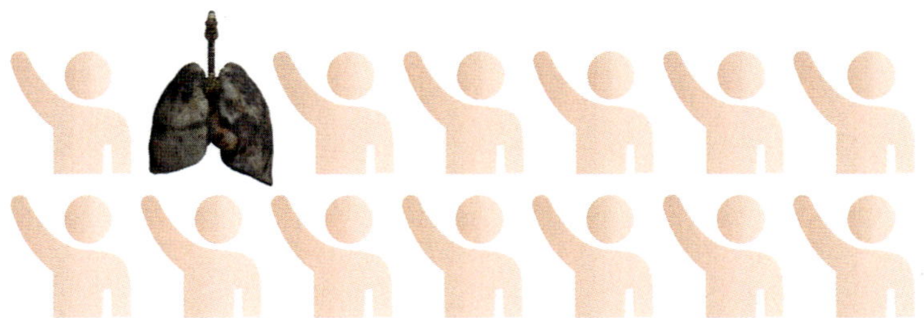

Figure 3
Cancer deaths in the United States

2.5 out of 10 cancer deaths are from lung cancer

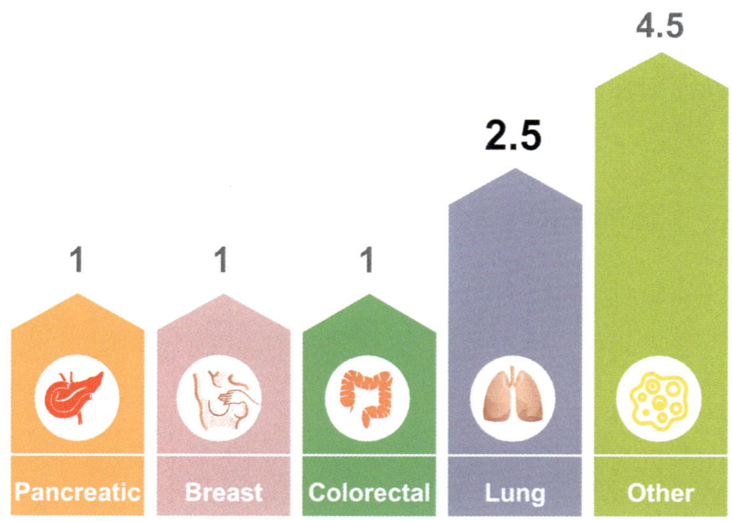

Types of lung cancer

Lung cancer has 2 main types:

1. Non-small cell lung cancer (NSCLC)

2. Small cell lung cancer (SCLC)

The most common type of lung cancer is NSCLC. It accounts for 8.5 out of 10 of all diagnosed lung cancers. NSCLC can be broken down into subtypes by looking at the cancer cells under a microscope. This is called histology.

Figure 4
Tumor in left lung

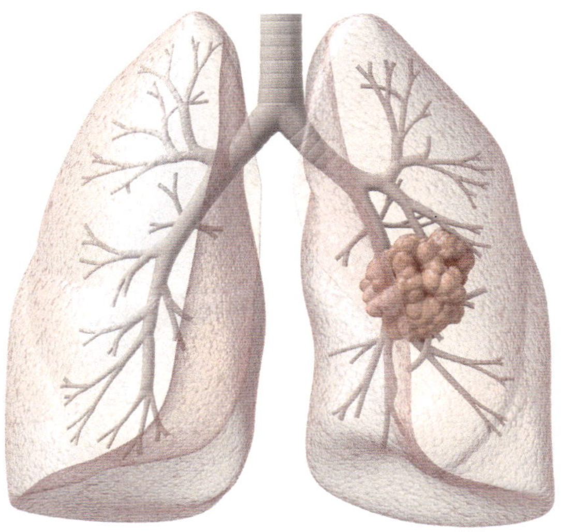

There are 3 subtypes of NSCLC:

- **Adenocarcinoma** starts in the cells that line the alveoli (small air sacs) in the lung. This is the most common subtype. About 4 out of 10 lung cancers are adenocarcinomas. **See Figure 4.**
- **Squamous cell (epidermoid) carcinoma** starts in the flat cells that line the inside of the airways in the lungs. About 3 out of 10 lung cancers are squamous cell carcinomas.
- **Large cell (undifferentiated) carcinoma** starts in large cells that can grow anywhere in the lungs. This accounts for 1.5 out of 10 lung cancers.

Other types of cancer can metastasize to the lungs, such as breast cancer. There are also less common types of cancer of the lung or chest. Lung screening may find non-cancerous conditions, tumors or benign diseases, and infections.

Review

- The lungs are a pair of organs in the chest that are vital to life.
- Lung cancer causes more deaths than any other cancer in both men and women.
- Lung cancer has 2 main types called NSCLC and SCLC.

2
Are you at risk?

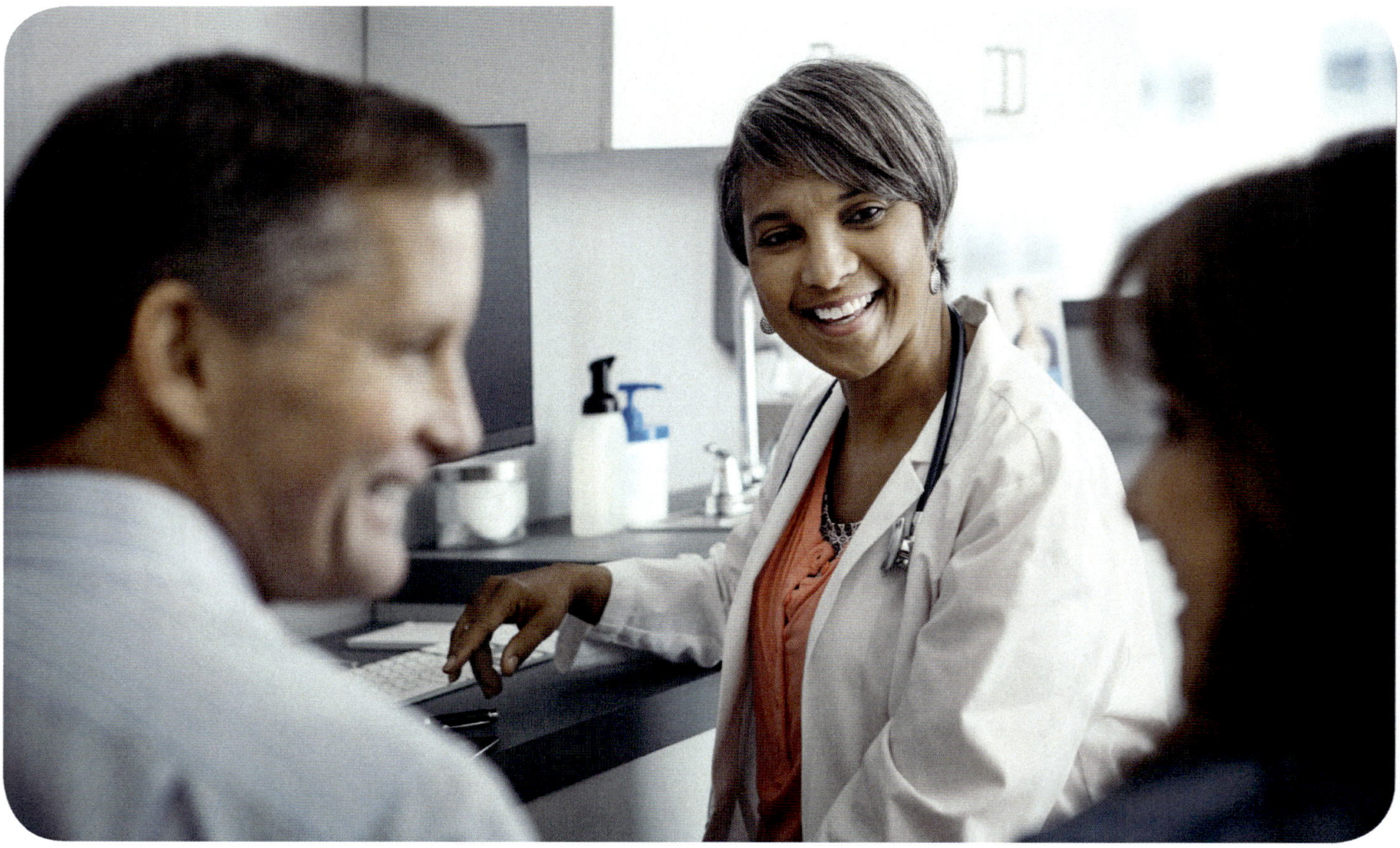

Some people are more likely than others to develop lung cancer. Anything that increases your chances of lung cancer is called a risk factor.

Risk factors for lung cancer

Risk factors can be activities that people do, things in the environment, or traits passed down from parents to children through genes. Genes are a set of instructions that tell new cells what to become (for example, lung, heart, and skin) and what to do (make hormones, absorb nutrients, and kill germs). If one or more risk factors applies to you, it does not mean you will get lung cancer. It just means lung cancer screening might be a good option for you. Some people who have none of the risk factors still get lung cancer. The known risk factors for lung cancer are listed in Guide 1.

Guide 1. Risk factors for lung cancer

Risk factors
Tobacco smoking
Contact with radon
Contact with asbestos or other cancer-causing agents
History of cancer
Famiy history of lung cancer
History of COPD or pulmonary fibrosis

Looking for help to quit smoking?

✓ Smokefree.gov
✓ BeTobaccoFree.gov

Tobacco smoking

Tobacco smoking is the biggest risk factor for lung cancer. It is a modifiable risk. This means you can take steps to change your risk by quitting smoking. Smoking tobacco causes lung cancer and accounts for 8.5 out of 10 lung cancer deaths. Smoking also increases the risk for other cancers, such as:

- head and neck
- bladder
- kidney
- pancreatic
- gastric
- cervical cancer
- acute myeloid leukemia

All smoking will increase your risk for lung cancer. Tobacco smoke has over 7,000 chemicals, and at least 70 of them cause cancer. The more you smoke, the higher your risk. If you quit smoking, your risk will decrease. Former smokers still have a higher risk of lung cancer than people who never smoked. Current or past tobacco smoking is a risk factor for lung cancer.

It is never too late to quit smoking. Smoking cessation counseling should be part of any lung cancer screening plan. Ask your doctor for support resources if you are interested in quitting smoking.

Second-hand smoke

Second-hand smoke is smoke from burning tobacco products, such as cigarettes, cigars, or pipes. It is also smoke that has been exhaled, or breathed out, by a person smoking. Second-hand smoke by itself is not considered a risk factor for lung cancer. Lung cancer screening is not recommended for people whose only risk factor is contact with second-hand smoke.

Radon

Radon is radioactive gas found in nature that can cause lung cancer. You cannot see or smell radon. Radon gas is given off by soil or rock and can enter buildings.

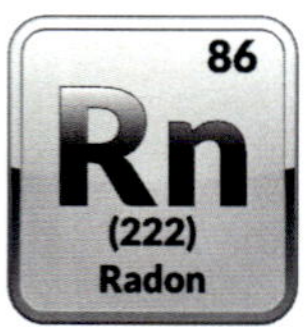

The risk for lung cancer may depend on how much radon is in the home and the number of years you have been exposed. For people who have been exposed to radon, the risk for lung cancer is higher if you smoke than for those who don't smoke.

Other cancer-causing agents

Besides radon, other cancer causing agents that target the lungs include the following:

- arsenic
- beryllium
- cadmium
- chromium
- nickel
- asbestos
- coal smoke
- soot
- silica
- diesel fumes

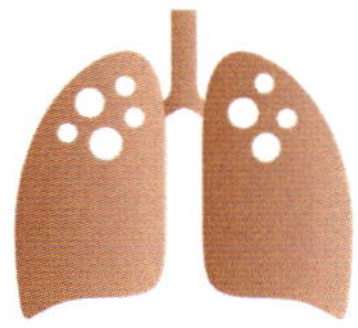

If you have been exposed to these agents, the risk for lung cancer is higher for smokers than for those who have never smoked.

History of cancer

If you've had other cancers, you might have an increased risk for lung cancer. The following increases your risk for new lung cancer:

- If you had small cell lung cancer
- If you had lymphoma
- If you had a smoking-related cancer, like bladder or head and neck cancer
- If you had chest radiation therapy or alkylating agent treatment
- If you were treated for Hodgkin lymphoma with alkylating agents or radiation therapy

It is never too late to stop smoking. Your future chances of smoking-related cancer may decrease if you were cured of a smoking-related lung cancer before and have since stopped smoking.

History of lung disease

A history of either chronic obstructive pulmonary disease (COPD) or pulmonary fibrosis increases your risk of lung cancer. In COPD the lung tissue is damaged causing a cough and too much mucus. Pulmonary fibrosis scars and thickens the tissue around and between the air sacs (alveoli) in your lungs making it hard to breathe. COPD includes emphysema and chronic bronchitis.

Family history of lung cancer

You have an increased risk of lung cancer if a close family relative has had lung cancer. Your risk is greater if your relative was diagnosed at a young age or if more than one relative has had lung cancer.

Hormone Replacement Therapy

Hormone replacement therapy (HRT) replaces natural hormones when the body does not make enough. It is unclear whether HRT affects the risk for lung cancer in women. More research is needed.

Review

- Anything that increases your chances of lung cancer is called a risk factor.
- Tobacco smoking is the biggest risk factor for lung cancer **(Figure 5)**.
- Ask your doctor for support resources that can help you quit smoking.

Figure 5
Tobacco smoking is the biggest risk factor for lung cancer

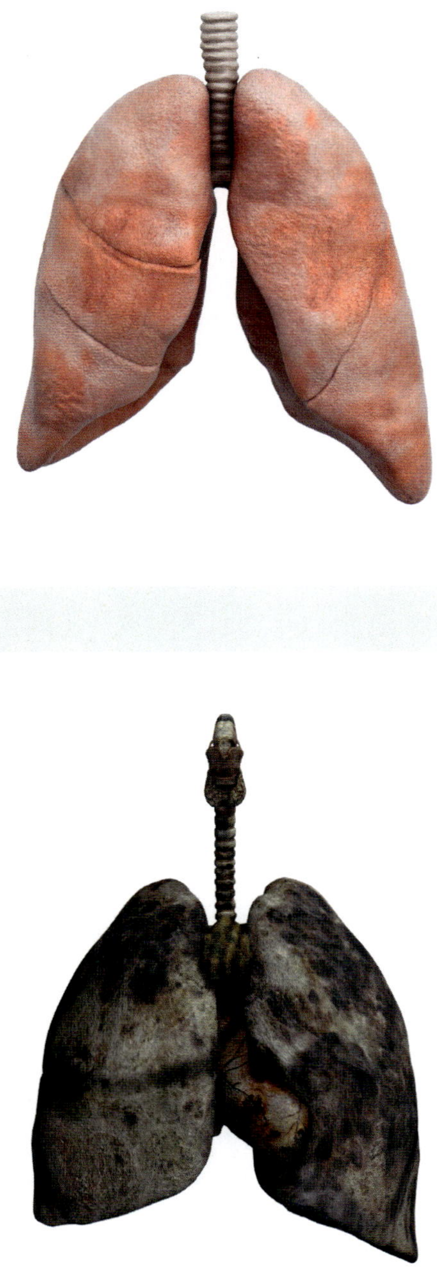

3
Should you start now?

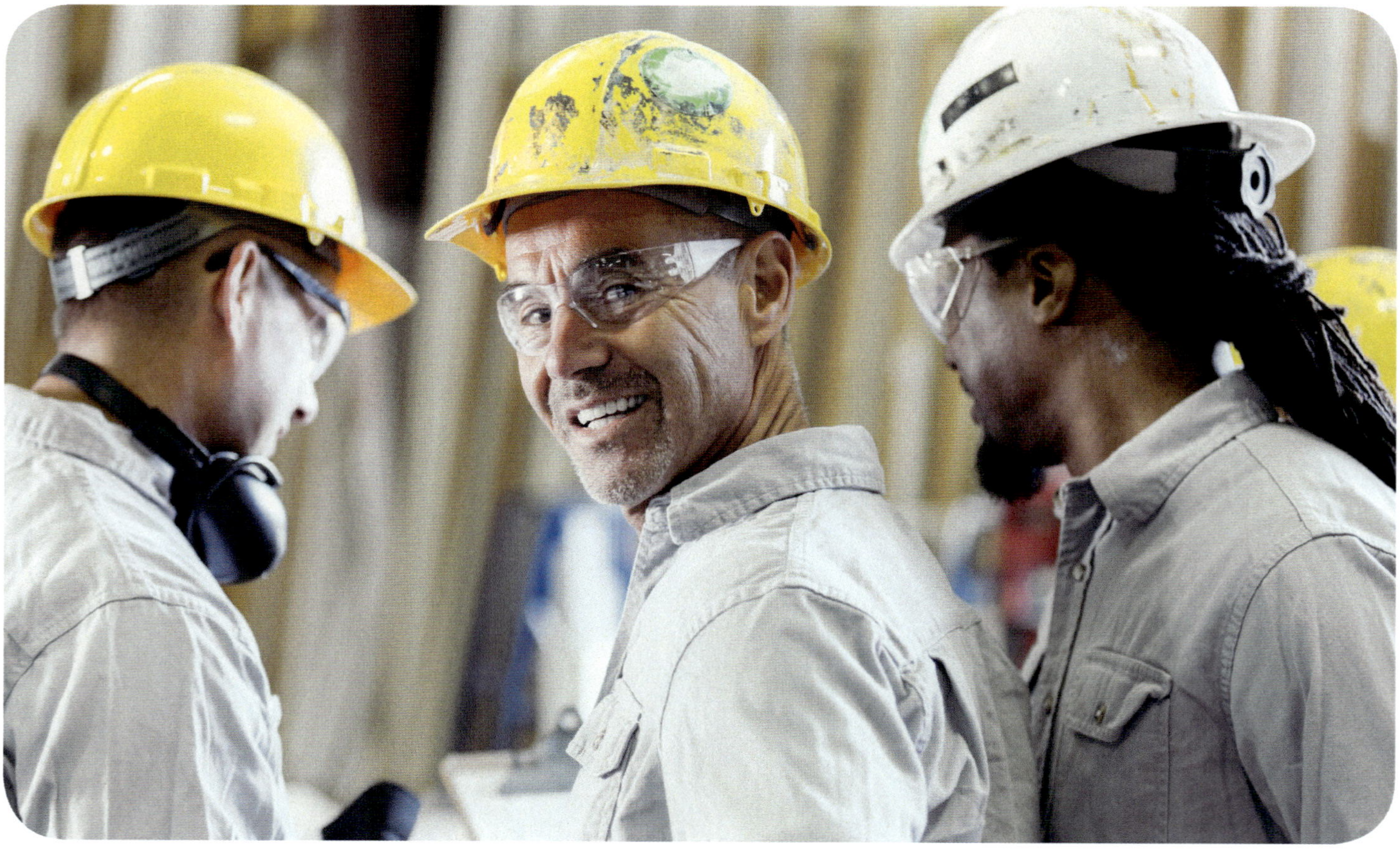

Start before you have symptoms

Screening can help find disease early, before symptoms occur. When disease is found early, it is more likely to be cured with treatment. The goal of lung cancer screening is to find lung cancer in people who are at a high risk for lung cancer. Treatment works best when started at an early stage of cancer, before there are symptoms. Most lung cancer is found after symptoms appear, when it may be too late to treat or cure.

Common symptoms of lung cancer are listed in Guide 2. See your doctor if you have these symptoms. Most often, these symptoms are caused by health problems other than lung cancer. Your health care provider may suggest other types of tests to check for cancer. If you have no symptoms of lung cancer, a screening program may be right for you.

Certain people are at risk for lung cancer. Tell your doctor about your medical history, family history, and work history. Let the doctor know if you smoked in the past and how many years it has been since you quit. Also, let the doctor know if you smoke now. Your doctor can then share the level of risk you have for lung cancer. The level of risk can be high, moderate, or low. If you are at high risk, learn about your screening options.

Screening test goals

- ✓ Finds cancer before symptoms occur
- ✓ Finds cancer at an early stage when it is easier to treat and cure
- ✓ Reduces chance of dying from cancer
- ✓ Has few false-positive and false-negative results

Guide 2. Symptoms of lung cancer

Symptoms of lung cancer	
Cough that lasts	Tiredness that lasts
Blood in mucus	Pneumonia
Shortness of breath	Hoarse voice
Wheezing	Pain when swallowing
Pain in chest area	Weight loss

Find out your level of risk

Guide 3 lists the criteria for high-, moderate-, and low-risk groups. There are two groups of people who are at high risk for lung cancer. Lung cancer screening is recommended for both high-risk groups.

As seen in Guide 3, the risk groups are divided by age and pack years of smoking. Smoking is based on pack years. A pack year is the number of packs of cigarettes you smoked every day multiplied by the number of years you smoked.

Guide 3. People at risk

Level of risk	Risk factors	Screening
High risk		
Group 1	• 55 to 77 years of age • 30 or more pack years of smoking and has quit within the past 14 years • Current smoker	Yearly screening is recommended
Group 2	• 50 years of age or older • 20 or more pack years of smoking • Other risk factors (other than second-hand smoke)	Yearly screening is recommended
Level of risk	**Risk factors**	**Screening**
Moderate risk	• 50 years of age or older • 20 or more pack years of smoking or contact with second-hand smoke • No other risk factors	Not recommended
Level of risk	**Risk factors**	**Screening**
Low risk	• 49 years of age or younger and/or • 19 or fewer pack years of smoking	Not recommended

Number of packs per day
x years of smoking
= Pack years

Example:

1.5 packs a day x 30 years = 45 pack years

Make a decision with your doctor

Lung cancer screening is based on your lung cancer risk factors. If you are in poor health or ill, screening might not be for you. Screening is for those who would seek treatment if lung cancer is found and who do not have other illnesses that would prevent treatment. People at high risk for lung cancer may benefit from low-dose computed tomography (LDCT) screening. Discuss with your doctor the risks and benefits of lung cancer screening. Together, decide whether or not to start lung cancer screening. This is called shared decision-making.

Shared decision-making is an important part of the doctor-patient relationship. It is where health care providers and patients work together to make decisions and choose tests and a treatment plan based on the risks and benefits. There is no "right" answer in a health care decision. Ask questions. Think about the different options. Decide what is best for you at the time. You can always change your mind.

Lung cancer screening should be part of a larger program of care and not done by itself. It is recommended that there be a team approach for lung cancer screening. Doctors or medical staff from different areas of medicine should work together to decide on a lung screening plan.

It takes skill to detect disease. For lung cancer screening, include specialists, when possible, from these areas in your program of care:

Thoracic (chest) radiology – a thoracic radiologist is an expert in reading test images for lung diseases

Pulmonary (lung) medicine – a pulmonologist is an expert in lung diseases

Thoracic surgery – a thoracic surgeon is an expert in operations within the chest

This team will:

- Assess your risk for lung cancer
- Review test results for signs of cancer

This team might:

- Repeat tests to see if there are any changes
- Order new tests
- Remove tissue from your body only if signs of cancer are present

Low-dose computed tomography test

An LDCT test is recommended as part of lung cancer screening. An LDCT uses small amounts of radiation and computer technology to take pictures of the inside of the body from different angles. The amount of radiation used is much lower than standard doses of a CT (computed tomography) scan. Contrast material should not be used for screening LDCT. A chest x-ray is not recommended for lung cancer screening. Lung cancer screening should not be used in place of quitting smoking.

Your initial or very first LDCT test is called the baseline LDCT. A first follow-up LDCT scan is done to compare to your baseline LDCT. You will have other follow-up LDCT tests every year or more often. The timing of your follow-up LDCTs are based on your risk factors for lung cancer and results of your previous LDCTs.

Risks

There are risks with any test. The LDCT might pick up abnormalities that look like cancer, but are not cancer. This error is called a false-positive result. With a false positive, you might have cancer-related tests, like a biopsy, only to find out you do not have cancer. The risk is that you might have tests that cost money and you do not need. Follow-up for a positive result is usually another LDCT test, not a biopsy. Given the number of false-positive results, you should discuss the risks and benefits of LDCT tests with your doctor before initial screening. See Guide 4.

A false negative is when your LDCT test results are clear, but you later find out you have lung cancer. A false negative might give you a false sense of comfort. It might cause you to ignore symptoms that might have led to more tests.

Limiting screening only to people who are at high risk for lung cancer helps to prevent unneeded testing. Shared decision-making with your doctor is the best approach in deciding whether to do LDCT lung screening. In shared decision-making, you and your doctor share information, weigh screening risks/benefits, and agree on the best plan.

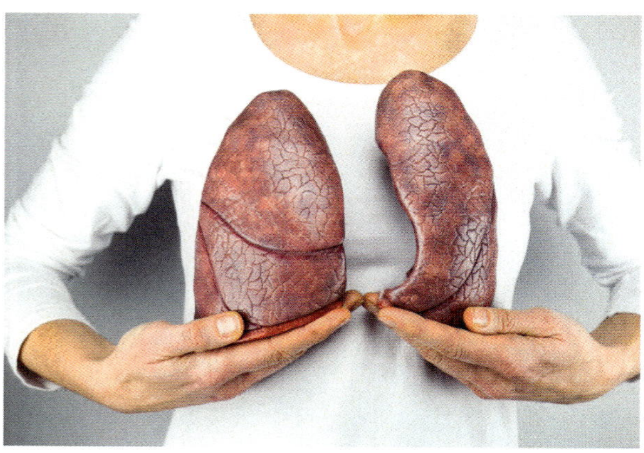

An LDCT is recommended as part of lung cancer screening.

Guide 4. Risks and benefits of LDCT lung cancer screening

Risks	Benefits
• Anxiety and worry waiting for test results	• Improves quality of life by finding cancer early • Lessens chance of death from lung cancer • Lessens chance of death from lung cancer treatment • Lessens chance of death from other diseases
• Test results could be wrong (false-positive or false-negative results)	• Follow-up and yearly tests help find cancer that might have been missed
• Screening costs money	• Screening saves money in the long run by catching disease early • If you are at high risk, screening cost might be covered or partly covered by insurance
• Finds tumors that can't be cured or doesn't find all lung cancers	• Finds other diseases like infection, COPD, coronary artery calcification, and kidney, adrenal, and liver lesions
• Contact with low levels of radiation (women are exposed to more radiation than men)	• Radiation levels are lower than in other tests
• Complications from follow-up tests • Overdiagnosis with unneeded testing or procedures	• Pre-screening of risk factors helps prevent unneeded tests • Only those at high risk are tested

Before the test

You should remove any metal objects on your body. These objects can affect the pictures taken of your lungs. The machine is large and has a tunnel in the middle. **See Figure 6**. During the test, you will lie on a table that moves through the tunnel. Pillows or straps may be used to keep you still during the test.

You will be alone in the room, but a CT technologist will operate the machine in a nearby room. The CT technologist can see you and the machine through a window. He or she will be able to hear and speak with you at all times.

During the test

The LDCT should be done by medical staff trained in screening for lung cancer. You will be asked to take a deep breath and hold it in for a few seconds while the pictures are being taken. This is done to make sure the images are of good quality and not blurry. As the machine takes pictures, you may hear buzzing, clicking, or whirring sounds. While it only takes seconds to take the pictures, the whole process takes about 20 to 30 minutes.

After the test

A radiologist, who is an expert at reading imaging tests, will look at and interpret your pictures. A report of the test results will be sent to your doctor. Together, you and your doctor will discuss the next steps based on the LDCT test results.

Review

- Lung cancer screening should start before cancer symptoms appear.
- Only people at high risk for lung cancer should consider a screening program.
- An LDCT test is recommended as part of lung cancer screening.

Figure 6
CT machine

A CT machine is large and has a tunnel in the middle. During the test, you will need to lie on a table that moves through the tunnel.

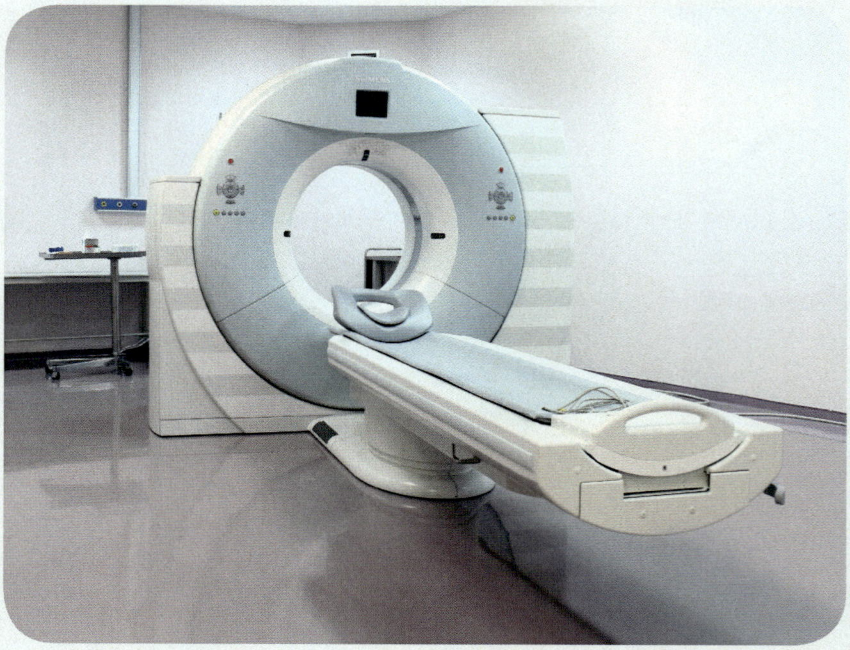

4 What happens after the first test?

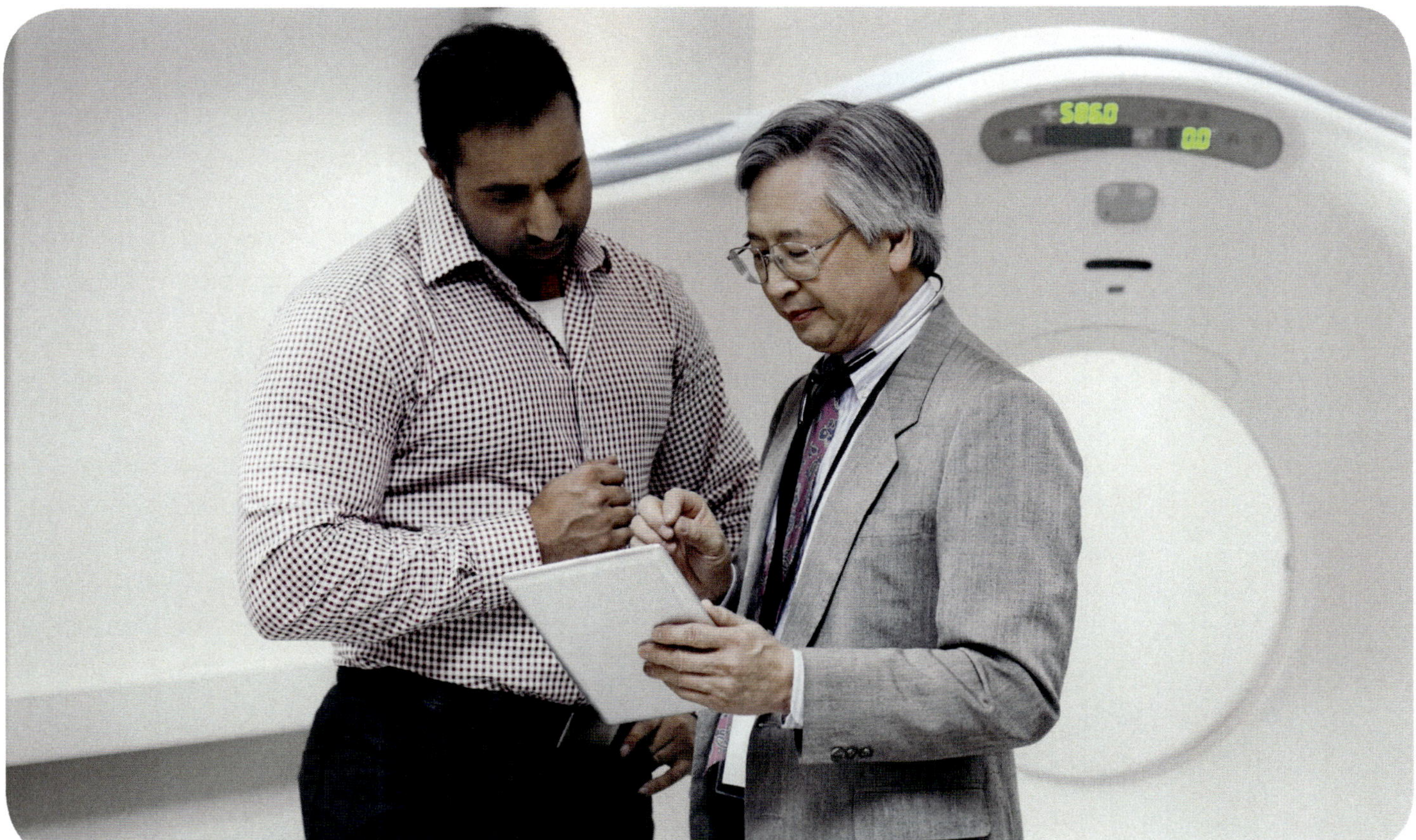

Types of lung nodules

Screening with LDCT is used to find nodules in the lungs. Nodules are small, round areas of tissue and are quite common. They appear as round, white shadows on an LDCT test. Nodules can be caused by cancer, infection, scar tissue, or other conditions. Most nodules are benign or not cancer. People can have one or more lung nodules found during the LDCT test. It takes a team of experts to decide if a nodule is cancer.

Features of the nodule

Nodules caused by cancer have specific traits.

- They aren't likely to have calcium buildup.
- They often have rough edges (called spiculations) and odd shapes.
- They often grow faster and are larger in size than nodules that are not cancer.
- Size and density are important.

If a lung nodule is new or has changed in size, shape, or appearance, your doctor may recommend further testing.

Size

Many of the nodules found on screening are small, about the size of a pea, and most of these nodules are not cancer. Nodules are measured in mm (millimeters) and are rounded to the nearest whole number. This letter "o" is about 2 mm long. A pea is about 5 mm.

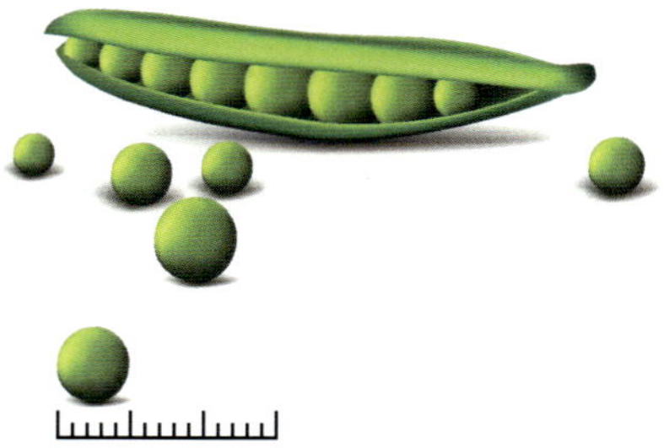

Nodules with cancer often grow faster and larger than those that are benign. There is an increased risk of cancer if a nodule is located in the upper lobes, especially the upper right lobe.

Density

Doctors assess how dense or solid a nodule is. This is a clue to whether or not the nodule is cancer. Density is how solid versus hazy a nodule looks on the LDCT pictures. A solid nodule has a higher density than a hazy one. Nodules are divided into groups based on density.

There are 2 main types of pulmonary (lung) nodules.

1. Solid nodules
    - **Solid nodules** look about as solid as your muscle does on an LDCT picture. This means they have a high density. Solid nodules are the most common type of nodule **(Figure 7)**.
2. Sub-solid nodules
    - **Part-solid nodules** or mixed solid nodules have both solid and non-solid (called ground-glass) areas. This means they have both high- and low-density areas. Part-solid nodules are mainly adenocarcinomas. Part-solid nodules have the greatest chance of being lung cancer.
    - **Non-solid nodules** look like a fuzzy or hazy cloud on an LDCT picture. These nodules are also called a "ground-glass opacity" (GGO) or a "ground-glass nodule" (GGN). Non-solid nodules are usually followed by more LDCT tests. Even if non-solid nodules are cancer, these are considered the kind of cancer that are unlikely to grow and spread.

Solid and part-solid nodules are more likely to be invasive and faster-growing cancers.

Chance of cancer

There is an increased concern for cancer in:

- Part-solid nodules with solid areas smaller than 5 mm that change in size
- Part-solid nodules with solid areas larger than 5 mm
- Pure non-solid nodules larger than 10 mm
- Pure non-solid nodules that change in size
- Sub-solid nodules with spiculations or with a bubbly, clustered look
- Solid lesions

All nodules will be closely monitored during lung cancer screening. You might have tests more often to track any changes in size, density, and appearance of nodules. If you have any questions about your nodules or the chance it might be cancer, talk to your doctor.

Figure 7
Nodule density

Solid and part-solid nodules are more likely to be invasive and faster-growing cancers

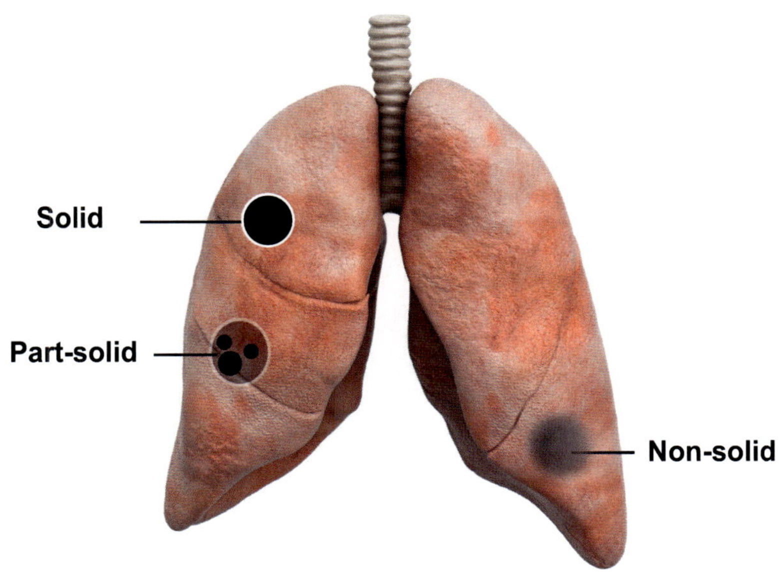

Overview of screening tests

Screening tests are repeated over time to see if a nodule may be cancer. See Guide 5. The schedule and type of screening test depend on whether there are changes in a nodule's size, density, or both. The first LDCT is called the baseline test. All future LDCT tests, called follow-ups, will be compared to this baseline test. The cutoff sizes differ for nodules found on the baseline LDCT when compared to new or growing nodules on follow-up LDCT scans. A radiologist will look for increases in size or density, or a change in shape. Such changes may be a sign of cancer.

Often, the use of one LDCT detects a nodule but it isn't clear whether or not the nodule is lung cancer. Sometimes, a chest CT scan with contrast or positron emission tomography (PET) scan might be ordered. A chest CT uses x-rays and computer technology to take images. The amount of radiation in a chest CT is higher than in an LDCT scan. A PET scan would check for disease throughout your body, and not just the chest area. Modern PET scanners are often called PET/CT scans.

PET scans

A PET scan may be used to look at a nodule that is found on a screening LDCT. A PET scan involves an injection of a small and safe amount of a radioactive sugar called glucose. After you get the glucose, pictures will be taken of the inside of your body. The doctor will look to see if the glucose is inside a lung nodule. Nodules that are cancer appear brighter or "hot" on the pictures. This happens because cancer cells use sugar more quickly than normal cells. However, very small nodules are not easily seen on PET. These nodules could be the size of a large pea or smaller. Cancers of that size don't use enough sugar to be detected.

Guide 5. Screening tests

Order of screening tests
Baseline screening LDCT
First follow-up screening LDCT
Follow-up or yearly screening LDCT
If needed, chest CT or PET/CT

Baseline LDCT

No lung nodules

If no lung nodules are found on the initial or baseline LDCT, then your next LDCT should be in 12 months. This would be your first follow-up LDCT. After that, you will continue to have LDCT tests every 12 months. Your doctor will look at your needs and decide how long to continue lung cancer screening.

Solid lung nodule

If a solid lung nodule is found during your baseline LDCT, the timing and type of your next test is shown in Guide 6. When and what type of test depends on the size of the solid lung nodule(s). A follow-up LDCT might be in 3, 6, or 12 months or you might have a chest CT with contrast and/or a PET/CT. A chest CT or PET/CT is often the next test for nodules with a concern for cancer. A biopsy would be done to confirm cancer.

Guide 6. Solid lung nodule on baseline LDCT

Size of solid lung nodule	Follow-up needed					
5 mm or smaller	LDCT in 12 months					
6 to 7 mm	LDCT in 6 months					
8 to 14 mm	LDCT in 3 months					
	Consider getting a PET/CT	Low concern for lung cancer	→	LDCT in 3 months		
		High concern for lung cancer	→	Biopsy or surgical excision		
15 mm or larger	Chest CT with contrast and/or PET/CT	Low concern for lung cancer	→	LDCT in 3 months		
		High concern for lung cancer	→	Biopsy or surgical excision	→	If no cancer, LDCT every 12 months until treatment is not an option If cancer, start treatment
Solid endobronchial nodule	LDCT in 1 month or less (after intense coughing)	→	If no result	→	Bronchoscopy	

If you have a solid lung nodule that is:

- 5 mm or smaller - your next LDCT should be in 12 months
- 6 to 7 mm - you should have a follow-up LDCT in 6 months
- 8 to 14 mm – you should have a follow-up LDCT in 3 months or consider a PET/CT
- 15 mm or larger – a chest CT and/or PET/CT scan is recommended

A nodule that is 15 mm or larger has the highest risk of cancer. Depending on the results of a chest CT and/or PET/CT, the next step might be to have a biopsy (sample the nodule) or surgical excision (remove the entire nodule) to check for cancer. If no cancer is found, your next LDCT should be in 12 months. If cancer is confirmed, you can start cancer treatment.

Solid endobronchial nodule

If a solid endobronchial nodule is found, your next LDCT will be in 1 month or less. This type of nodule can grow in the large breathing tubes (bronchi) that lead to the lungs. Just before your LDCT, the technician will ask you to cough vigorously. If there is no result from the LDCT, then a bronchoscopy should be done. A bronchoscopy is when a long, thin camera is guided into the airway to look at or remove tissue.

If there is high concern for cancer, the next step would be to have a biopsy (remove one or more samples of tissue) or surgical excision (remove the entire nodule) to check for cancer. This is done by looking at the cells under a microscope. If no cancer is found, your next LDCT should be in 12 months. If cancer is confirmed, you can start cancer treatment.

Part-solid lung nodule

In a part-solid nodule, both the whole nodule and the solid area are measured. See Guide 7.

If you have a part-solid lung nodule in a baseline LDCT that is:

- 5 mm or smaller - your next LDCT should be in 12 months
- 6 mm or larger with a solid part of 5 mm or smaller – your next LDCT should be in 6 months
- 6 mm or larger with a solid part of 6 to 7 mm – your next LDCT should be in 3 months or you should consider a PET/CT
- Solid part of 8 mm or larger – get a chest CT and/or a PET/CT

The timing of your next LDCT screening test is based on both the size of the whole nodule and size of the solid part. For those part-solid nodules with a solid part of 8 mm or larger, a PET/CT is recommended. For those where the solid part is 6 to 7 mm, consider getting a PET/CT. PET/CT scans have trouble measuring nodules that are 8 mm or less or are in certain locations of the lung. This is why your team will consider other factors before ordering a PET/CT when the part-solid nodule is in this size range.

Non-solid lung nodule

Your next LDCT test is based on the results of the baseline LDCT. Many non-solid nodules can be followed-up with an LDCT every 12 months. See Guide 8. You should have an LDCT in 6 months for a non-solid lung nodule that is 20 mm or larger. An olive or a cherry is about 20 mm.

Non-solid nodules may be cancer, but they may also be small areas of infection or inflammation. Large nodules are more likely to be cancer than small nodules. If a non-solid nodule develops a solid part on a future LDCT, this is a sign it could be cancer. The LDCT test will focus on taking good pictures of the solid part of any part-solid nodule.

Guide 7. Part-solid lung nodule on baseline LDCT

<table>
<tr><th colspan="2">Size of part-solid lung nodule</th><th colspan="4">Follow-up needed</th></tr>
<tr><td colspan="2">5 mm or smaller</td><td colspan="4">LDCT in 12 months</td></tr>
<tr><td rowspan="2">6 mm or larger with</td><td>Solid part 5 mm or smaller</td><td colspan="4">LDCT in 6 months</td></tr>
<tr><td>Solid part 6 to 7 mm</td><td colspan="4">LDCT in 3 months
or
Consider getting PET/CT</td></tr>
<tr><td colspan="2" rowspan="2">Solid part 8 mm or larger</td><td rowspan="2">Chest CT with contrast
and/or
PET/CT</td><td>Low concern for lung cancer</td><td colspan="2">➔ LDCT in 3 months</td></tr>
<tr><td>High concern for lung cancer</td><td>➔ Biopsy or surgical excision</td><td>➔ If no cancer, LDCT every 12 months until treatment is not an option
If cancer, start treatment</td></tr>
</table>

Guide 8. Non-solid lung nodule on baseline LDCT

Size of non-solid lung nodule	Follow-up needed
19 mm or smaller	LDCT in 12 months
20 mm or larger	LDCT in 6 months

Follow-up or yearly LDCT

Your doctor will compare your first follow-up LDCT to the baseline LDCT test. Then, he or she will decide when your next follow-up test will occur. Usually your next LDCT will be in 12 months, but you might have an LDCT in 3 or 6 months or you might have a chest CT or PET/CT as suggested by your doctor. These decisions are based on your test results. If you have a new or growing nodule, it might be tested more often. The nodule size and density are also factors.

New lung nodule on follow-up

Inflammation or infection might be the reason behind a new nodule found on a follow-up or yearly LDCT. If your doctor thinks this is the reason, then a follow-up LDCT will be in 1 to 3 months. During this time, your doctor may treat the infection or inflammation. Ongoing LDCT follow-up tests depend on if the infection or inflammation does or does not go away. If you have any questions, ask your doctor. See Guide 9.

It is important to have yearly LDCT tests

✓ Screening helps find disease early when it is easier to treat and cure

Guide 9. New nodule on follow-up or yearly LDCT

Results	Next LDCT	How does the nodule look?		Follow-up needed
Possible infection or inflammation	LDCT in 1 to 3 months	Getting better	➔	LDCT in 3 to 6 months
		Better	➔	LDCT in 12 months
		Not getting better or it is growing	➔	Next test depends on size and type of nodule

Solid lung nodule on follow-up

The timing of the next LDCT test is based on the size of the solid nodule and whether is it new or growing. See Guide 10. Your doctor will compare the results from all of your tests to decide when you should have the next test. A new, smaller solid nodule might be tested sooner than a larger nodule that has not changed over time. Sometimes, additional tests such as a chest CT or PET/CT scan are recommended.

Guide 10. Solid lung nodule on follow-up or yearly LDCT

Results	Size of lung nodule		Follow-up needed
No change on follow-up LDCT	7 mm or smaller	➔	LDCT in 12 months
	8 to 14 mm	➔	LDCT in 6 months
	15 mm or larger	➔	LDCT in 6 months or PET/CT
Results	**Size of lung nodule**		**Follow-up needed**
No change on yearly LDCT	No change on yearly LDCT	➔	LDCT in 12 months
Results	**Size of lung nodule**		**Follow-up needed**
New nodule	3 mm or smaller	➔	LDCT in 12 months
	4 to 5 mm	➔	LDCT in 6 months
	6 to 7 mm	➔	LDCT in 3 months
	8 mm or larger	➔	Chest CT with contrast or PET/CT
Results	**Size of lung nodule**		**Follow-up needed**
Growing nodule - larger than 1.5 mm	7 mm or smaller	➔	LDCT in 3 months
	8 mm or larger	➔	Chest CT with contrast or PET/CT

A chest CT or PET/CT scan might be ordered when there is concern for cancer. If there is a high concern for cancer, a biopsy or surgical excision of the solid lung nodule can confirm cancer. If cancer is confirmed, then treatment will start. If no cancer, then you will have LDCT tests every 12 months.

Part-solid lung nodule on follow-up

In a part-solid nodule, both the whole nodule and the solid part are measured.

The timing of your next LDCT screening test is based on the following:

- size of the whole nodule and size of the solid part
- if it is a new nodule
- if it is a growing nodule
- if there was no change from an earlier LDCT

If the part-solid lung nodule had no change on the LDCT done last year and is 5 mm or smaller, your next LDCT should be in 12 months. For those part-solid nodules that are new, or are growing and are 6 mm or larger, your next LDCT depends on the size of both the whole nodule and the solid part. See Guide 11 for more information on the timing of your next LDCT for part-solid nodules.

You will have further testing based on the nodule size and concern for cancer. If there is a low concern for cancer, you should get an LDCT in 3 or 6 months. If there is a high concern for cancer, you should have a biopsy or surgical excision. This is done instead of waiting to see if anything changes over time. A biopsy or surgical excision of the nodule can confirm if cancer is present.

In a part-solid nodule, both the whole nodule and the solid part are measured.

Guide 11. Part-solid lung nodule on follow-up or yearly LDCT

Results	Size of lung nodule		Follow-up needed
No change on follow-up LDCT	5 mm or smaller	➡	LDCT in 12 months
	6 mm or larger with 6 to 7 mm solid part	➡	LDCT in 6 months
	6 mm or larger with 8 mm or larger solid part	➡	LDCT in 6 months or PET/CT

Results	Size of lung nodule		Follow-up needed
No change on yearly LDCT	No change on yearly LDCT	➡	LDCT in 12 months

Results	Size of lung nodule		Follow-up needed
New nodule	5 mm or smaller	➡	LDCT in 6 months

Results	Size of lung nodule		Follow-up needed
Growing nodule with solid part larger than 1.5 mm or new nodule	6 mm or larger with growing solid part 3 mm or smaller	➡	LDCT in 3 months
	4 mm or larger solid part	➡	Chest CT with contrast and/or PET/CT

Non-solid lung nodule on follow-up

If a non-solid nodule has disappeared or gotten smaller between tests, there is a chance it was a small infection and not cancer. See Guide 12 for more information on the timing of your next LDCT for non-solid nodules.

- For a new or stable (not growing) 19 mm or smaller non-solid nodule, your next LDCT should be in 12 months.
- For a new or stable 20 mm or larger non-solid nodule, your next LDCT should be in 6 months.
- If a nodule has grown or become more solid, it may be cancer. Because of this concern, an LDCT should be in 6 months or your doctor will consider a biopsy or surgical excision.

Guide 12. Non-solid lung nodule on follow-up or yearly LDCT

Results	Size of non-solid lung nodule		Follow-up needed
New nodule	19 mm or smaller	➔	LDCT in 12 months
	20 mm or larger		LDCT in 6 months
Results	**Size of non-solid lung nodule**		**Follow-up needed**
Stable nodule	19 mm or smaller	➔	LDCT in 12 months
	20 mm or larger		LDCT in 6 months
Results	**Size of non-solid lung nodule**		**Follow-up needed**
Growing nodule (growth of more than 1. 5 mm)	19 mm or smaller	➔	LDCT in 6 months
	20 mm or larger	➔	LDCT in 6 months or Consider biopsy or surgical excision

Biopsy

A biopsy is the removal of tissue or a group of cells by a surgeon. A biopsy looks for signs of cancer in your cells. To test for cancer, tissue from the lung nodule is removed from your body. The tissue is sent to a lab and examined under a microscope by a pathologist. Enough tissue needs to be removed in order to properly test the sample.

A biopsy removes small samples of tissue. Surgery or surgical excision removes the entire nodule for testing. Since a biopsy only removes a very small piece of the nodule, the results could be wrong. There may be cancer cells in another part of the nodule. Your lung cancer screening team may suggest surgery to remove the whole nodule if your risk for cancer is high. Your doctor may suggest another biopsy, surgery, or more testing if the first biopsy shows no cancer, but cancer is suspected.

Biopsy sample

If cancer cells are found in the biopsy or surgical tissue, read the *NCCN Patient Guidelines: Lung Cancer®*. Treatment options are recommended for every stage of lung cancer.

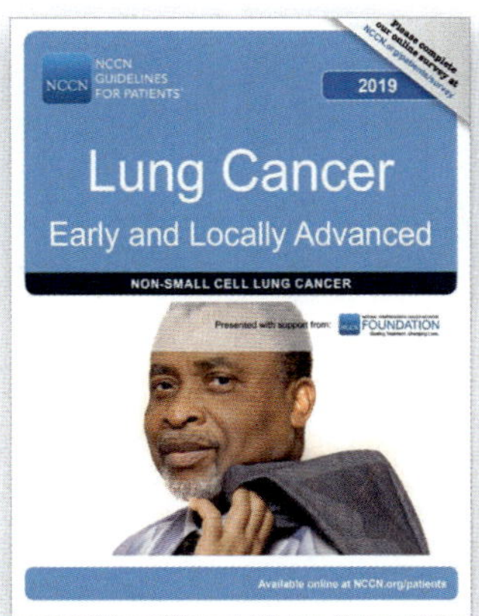

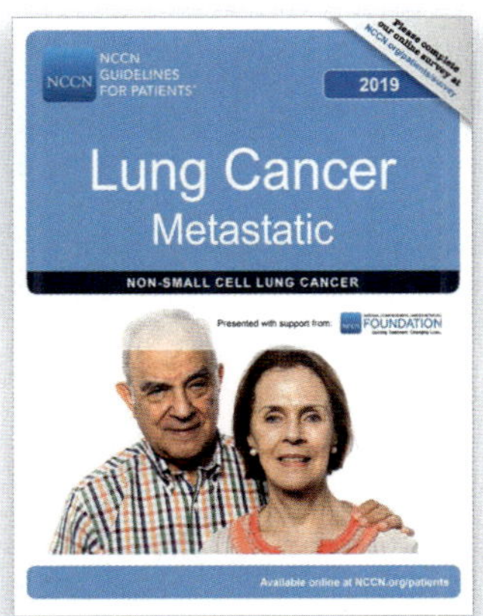

When no cancer is found in the biopsy or surgical tissue, yearly screening is suggested. Sometimes a sample of tissue from the biopsy does not have enough cells to check for cancer or may be abnormal but not cancer. Ask your doctor if you have any questions about your test results and when your next test might be.

Review

- Many people have lung nodules. Nodules can be caused by cancer, infections, scar tissue, or other conditions.
- Often, screening tests are repeated over time to assess if a nodule may be cancer.
- The schedule and type of screening test depend on whether there are changes in a nodule's size, density, or both.

5
What questions do you have?

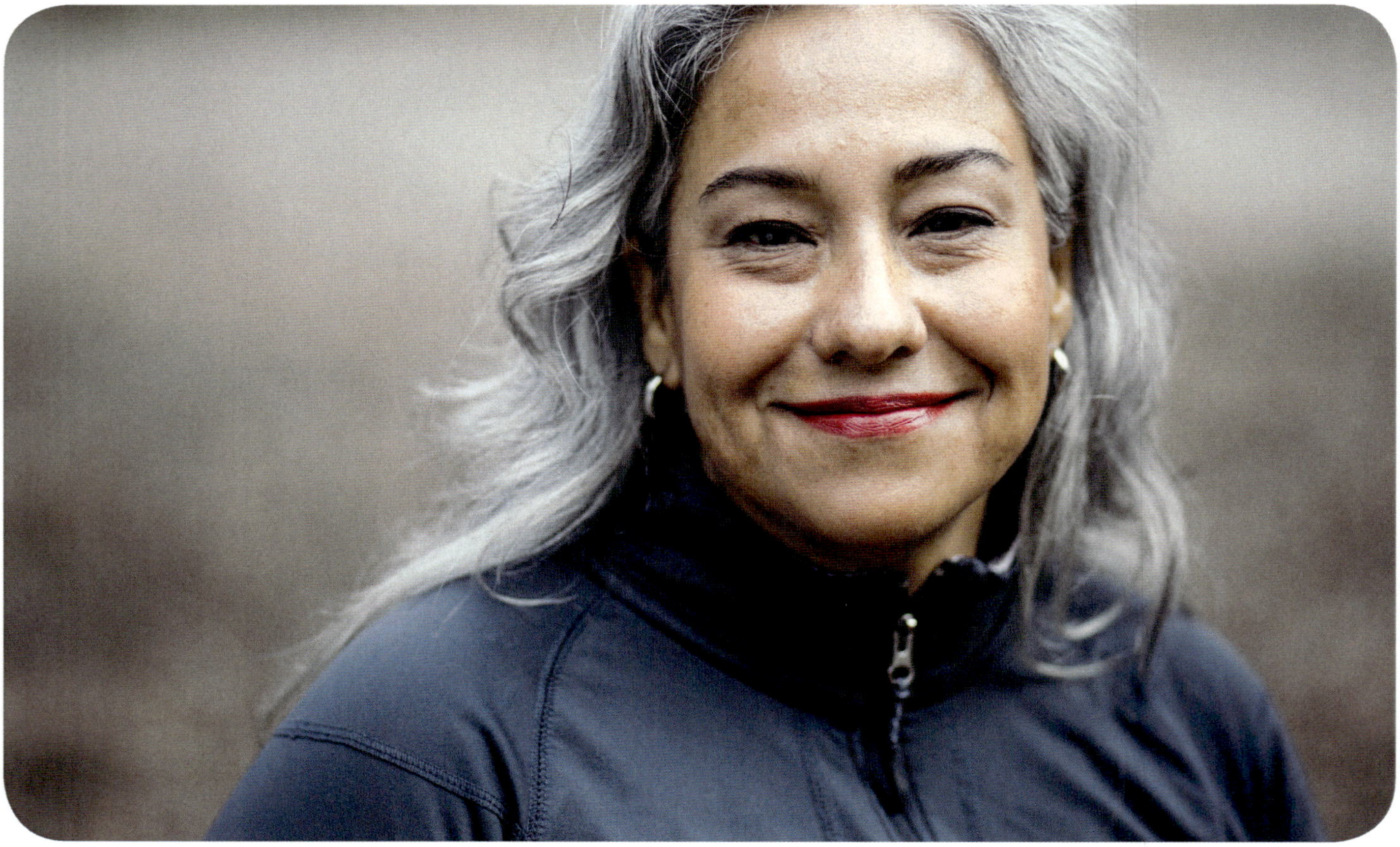

Talk with your health care provider about your risks for lung cancer. Together, decide if starting a lung cancer screening program now is right for you.

If you decide to move forward, most testing sites and insurance companies require a doctor's prescription before you have an LDCT test. Check with your insurance company to make sure you have met all of its requirements in order to be tested for lung cancer. For instance, the Centers for Medicare & Medicaid Services (CMS) requires not only that you meet certain risk factors, but that you receive counseling and participate in shared decision-making with your health care provider. This must be done before lung cancer screening. If you have questions, ask your health care provider.

Screening plan

In a good screening plan the benefits will outweigh the risks. Before starting a screening plan, talk with your doctor about all of the possible benefits and risks of the plan.

Benefits should include:

- Better survival and quality of life
- Less testing and treatment
- Support to quit smoking
- Lower costs

Questions to ask your doctors

It is important to learn all you can about screening so you can engage in shared decision-making with your doctor. It is a good idea to get your questions ready before your visit and repeat back what answers you hear. You can also think about bringing a family member or friend to the visit who can take notes and ask questions.

The following questions are suggestions to learn more about lung cancer screening. Feel free to use these questions or come up with your own questions for your doctor.

Questions about screening

1. Should I be screened for lung cancer?
2. What screening plan do you recommend for me? Why?
3. What are the benefits and risks of this screening plan?
4. Do you use LDCT for screening? Where can I find a testing site?
5. What type of smoking cessation program and counseling do you suggest for me?
6. Do you have a team of experts who are dedicated to lung cancer screening? Do they include board-certified pulmonologists, thoracic surgeons, and thoracic radiologists?
7. What do I have to do to prepare for screening?
8. How long will screening take?
9. How soon will I know the results? Who will explain them to me?
10. What type of nodule(s) do I have? What does this mean?

Questions about biopsies

1. What type of biopsy will I have?
2. What are the risks with this type of biopsy?
3. When will I know the results and who will explain them to me?

Review

- Find a screening site that provides high-quality care and specializes in LDCT tests.
- Decide on a screening plan that has many benefits and few risks.
- Ask your doctor questions. Getting the right information is vital to making decisions about screening.

Websites

American Cancer Society
cancer.org/cancer/lung-cancer.html

American Lung Association
lung.org

Bonnie J. Addario Lung Cancer Foundation
lungcancerfoundation.org

Caring Ambassadors Program, Inc.
lungcancercap.org

Dusty Joy Foundation (LiveLung)
LiveLung.org

Free ME from Lung Cancer
freeMEfromLungCancer.org

Lung Cancer Action Network (LungCAN)
LungCAN.org

Lung Cancer Alliance
lungcanceralliance.org

Lung Cancer Circle of Hope
lungcancercircleofhope.org

Lung Cancer Initiative of North Carolina
lungcancerinitiativenc.org

Lung Cancer Research Foundation
lcrf.org

LUNGevity Foundation
LUNGevity.org

National Cancer Institute (NCI)
cancer.gov/types/lung

National Coalition for Cancer Survivorship
canceradvocacy.org/toolbox

NCCN for Patients®
nccn.org/patients

Smoking cessation (help to quit smoking)
smokefree.gov
BeTobaccoFree.gov

Words to know

alkylating agent
A type of cancer-killing drug.

arsenic
A very toxic metallic chemical.

asbestos
A mineral fiber used in housing and commercial materials.

baseline test
A starting point to which future tests are compared.

benign
Tissue without cancer cells.

beryllium
A hard, gray metallic chemical.

biopsy
Removal of small amounts of tissue or fluid to be tested for disease.

bladder
An organ that holds and expels urine from the body.

board certified
A status to identify doctors who finished training in a specialized field of medicine.

bronchoscopy
Use of a long, thin camera guided down the mouth into the lungs.

cadmium
A heavy metallic chemical.

calcium
A mineral found in body tissues.

cancer screening
The use of tests to find cancer before signs of cancer appear.

chromium
A hard, semi-gray metallic chemical.

chronic obstructive pulmonary disease (COPD)
Trouble with breathing due to lung damage or too much mucus.

computed tomography (CT)
A test that combines many x-rays to make pictures of the inside of the body.

curative treatment
A medicine that cures disease or symptoms.

diesel fumes
Gases from fuel that is thick, heavy, and made from crude oil.

early stage
Cancer that has had little or no growth into nearby tissues.

electromagnetic
A force that attracts or repels and is produced by an electric current.

follow-up test
A close watch by doctors of possible cancer using tests.

genes
Instructions in cells for making and controlling cells.

ground-glass nodule (GGN)
A small mass of non-solid lung cells with low density.

ground-glass opacity (GGO)
A small mass of non-solid lung cells with low density.

Hodgkin lymphoma
A cancer of white blood cells.

infection
An illness caused by germs.

inflammation
Redness, heat, pain, and swelling from injury or infection.

lobe
A clearly seen division in the lungs.

low-dose computed tomography (LDCT)
A test that uses little amounts of radiation to make pictures of the inside of the body.

lung
An organ in the body made of airways and air sacs.

lymph node
A small group of disease-fighting cells.

millimeters (mm)
A unit of length measuring one thousandth of a meter.

mucus
A sticky, thick liquid that moisturizes or lubricates.

NCCN®
National Comprehensive Cancer Network

nickel
A silvery-white metal.

nodule
A small mass of tissue.

non-solid nodule
A small mass of tissue of low density.

non-small cell lung cancer (NSCLC)
A cancer of lung cells that are not small.

pack years
The number of cigarette packs smoked every day multiplied by the number of years of smoking.

part-solid nodule
A small mass of tissue with areas of low and high density.

positron emission tomography (PET)
A test that uses radioactive material to see the shape and function of body parts.

pulmonary fibrosis
Major scarring of lung tissue.

pulmonologist
A doctor who's an expert in lung diseases.

radiologist
A doctor who's an expert in reading imaging tests.

radon
A gas without odor, taste, or color that is made from uranium as it decays.

risk factor
Something that increases the chance of getting a disease.

scar tissue
Supportive fibers formed to heal a wound.

second-hand smoke
Inhaled smoke from a lit smoking product or that was exhaled by a smoker.

silica
A natural mineral mostly found in sand.

small cell lung cancer (SCLC)
A cancer of small, round lung cells.

solid nodule
A small mass of tissue of high density.

surgical excision
Entire nodule is removed during surgery using a sharp knife (scalpel).

thoracic surgeon
A doctor who's an expert in surgery within the chest.

tumor
An abnormal mass of cells.

wheezing
A coarse, whistling sound while breathing.

NCCN Contributors

This patient guide is based on the NCCN Clinical Practice Guidelines in Oncology (NCCN Guidelines®) for Lung Cancer Screening. It was adapted, reviewed, and published with help from the following people:

Dorothy A. Shead, MS
Director, Patient Information Operations

Laura J. Hanisch, PsyD
Medical Writer/Patient Information Specialist

Erin Vidic, MA
Medical Writer

Rachael Clarke
Senior Medical Copyeditor

Tanya Fischer, MEd, MSLIS
Medical Writer

Kim Williams
Creative Services Manager

Susan Kidney
Design Specialist

The NCCN Clinical Practice Guidelines in Oncology (NCCN Guidelines®) for Lung Cancer Screening Version 1.2020 were developed by the following NCCN Panel Members:

Douglas E. Wood, MD/Chair
University of Washington/ Seattle Cancer Care Alliance

Ella A. Kazerooni, MD, MS/Vice Chair
University of Michigan Rogel Cancer Center

*Scott L. Baum, MD
The University of Tennessee Health Science Center

George A. Eapen, MD
The University of Texas MD Anderson Cancer Center

David S. Ettinger, MD
The Sidney Kimmel Comprehensive Cancer Center at Johns Hopkins

J. Scott Ferguson, MD
University of Wisconsin Carbone Cancer Center

Lifang Hou, MD, PhD
Robert H. Lurie Comprehensive Cancer Center of Northwestern University

Donald Klippenstein, MD
Moffitt Cancer Center

Rohit Kumar, MD
Fox Chase Cancer Center

Rudy P. Lackner, MD
Fred & Pamela Buffett Cancer Center

*Lorriana E. Leard, MD
UCSF Helen Diller Family Comprehensive Cancer Center

Inga T. Lennes, MD, MPH, MBA
Massachusetts General Hospital Cancer Center

Ann N.C. Leung, MD
Stanford Comprehensive Cancer Center

Pierre P. Massion, MD
Vanderbilt-Ingram Cancer Center

Peter Mazzone, MD, MPH
Case Comprehensive Cancer Center University Hospitals Seidman Cancer Center and Cleveland Clinic Taussig Cancer Institute

Robert E. Merritt, MD
The Ohio State University Comprehensive Cancer Center - James Cancer Hospital and Solove Research Institute

David E. Midthun, MD
Mayo Clinic Cancer Center

Mark Onaitis, MD
UC San Diego Moores Cancer Center

Sudhakar Pipavath, MD
University of Washington/ Seattle Cancer Care Alliance

*Christie Pratt, DHSc, MA
Moffitt Cancer Center

Varun Puri, MD, MSCI
Siteman Cancer Center at Barnes-Jewish Hospital and Washington University School of Medicine

Chakravarthy Reddy, MD
Huntsman Cancer Institute at the University of Utah

*Mary E. Reid, PhD
Roswell Park Cancer Institute

Arnold J. Rotter, MD
City of Hope National Medical Center

Peter B. Sachs, MD
University of Colorado Cancer Center

Jacob Sands, MD
Dana-Farber/Brigham and Women's Cancer Center

Matthew B. Schabath, PhD
Moffitt Cancer Center

Lynn Tanoue, MD
Yale Cancer Center/Smilow Cancer Hospital

Betty C. Tong, MD, MHS
Duke Cancer Institute

William D. Travis, MD
Memorial Sloan Kettering Cancer Center

Anil Vachani, MD
Abramson Cancer Center at the University of Pennsylvania

*Benjamin Wei, MD
O'Neal Comprehensive Cancer Center at UAB

Stephen C. Yang, MD
The Sidney Kimmel Comprehensive Cancer Center at Johns Hopkins

NCCN Staff

Kristina M. Gregory, RN, MSN, OCN
Vice President/Clinical Information Operations

Miranda Hughes, PhD
Oncology Scientist/Senior Medical Writer

* Reviewed this patient guide.
For disclosures, visit www.nccn.org/about/disclosure.aspx.

NCCN Cancer Centers

Abramson Cancer Center
at the University of Pennsylvania
Philadelphia, Pennsylvania
800.789.7366
pennmedicine.org/cancer

Fred & Pamela Buffett Cancer Center
Omaha, Nebraska
800.999.5465
nebraskamed.com/cancer

Case Comprehensive Cancer Center/
University Hospitals Seidman Cancer
Center and Cleveland Clinic Taussig
Cancer Institute
Cleveland, Ohio
800.641.2422 • UH Seidman Cancer Center
uhhospitals.org/seidman
866.223.8100 • CC Taussig Cancer Institute
my.clevelandclinic.org/services/cancer
216.844.8797 • Case CCC
case.edu/cancer

City of Hope National Medical Center
Los Angeles, California
800.826.4673
cityofhope.org

Dana-Farber/Brigham and
Women's Cancer Center
Massachusetts General Hospital
Cancer Center
Boston, Massachusetts
877.332.4294
dfbwcc.org
massgeneral.org/cancer

Duke Cancer Institute
Durham, North Carolina
888.275.3853
dukecancerinstitute.org

Fox Chase Cancer Center
Philadelphia, Pennsylvania
888.369.2427
foxchase.org

Huntsman Cancer Institute
at the University of Utah
Salt Lake City, Utah
877.585.0303
huntsmancancer.org

Fred Hutchinson Cancer
Research Center/Seattle
Cancer Care Alliance
Seattle, Washington
206.288.7222 • seattlecca.org
206.667.5000 • fredhutch.org

The Sidney Kimmel Comprehensive
Cancer Center at Johns Hopkins
Baltimore, Maryland
410.955.8964
hopkinskimmelcancercenter.org

Robert H. Lurie Comprehensive
Cancer Center of Northwestern
University
Chicago, Illinois
866.587.4322
cancer.northwestern.edu

Mayo Clinic Cancer Center
Phoenix/Scottsdale, Arizona
Jacksonville, Florida
Rochester, Minnesota
800.446.2279 • Arizona
904.953.0853 • Florida
507.538.3270 • Minnesota
www.mayoclinic.org/cancercenter

Memorial Sloan Kettering
Cancer Center
New York, New York
800.525.2225
mskcc.org

Moffitt Cancer Center
Tampa, Florida
800.456.3434
moffitt.org

The Ohio State University
Comprehensive Cancer Center -
James Cancer Hospital and
Solove Research Institute
Columbus, Ohio
800.293.5066
cancer.osu.edu

O'Neal Comprehensive
Cancer Center at UAB
Birmingham, Alabama
800.822.0933
uab.edu/onealcancercenter/

Roswell Park Comprehensive
Cancer Center
Buffalo, New York
877.275.7724
roswellpark.org

Siteman Cancer Center at Barnes-
Jewish Hospital and Washington
University School of Medicine
St. Louis, Missouri
800.600.3606
siteman.wustl.edu

St. Jude Children's
Research Hospital
The University of Tennessee
Health Science Center
Memphis, Tennessee
888.226.4343 • stjude.org
901.683.0055 • westclinic.com

Stanford Cancer Institute
Stanford, California
877.668.7535
cancer.stanford.edu

UC San Diego Moores Cancer Center
La Jolla, California
858.657.7000
cancer.ucsd.edu

UCSF Helen Diller Family
Comprehensive Cancer Center
San Francisco, California
800.689.8273
cancer.ucsf.edu

University of Colorado Cancer Center
Aurora, Colorado
720.848.0300
coloradocancercenter.org

University of Michigan
Rogel Cancer Center
Ann Arbor, Michigan
800.865.1125
mcancer.org

The University of Texas
MD Anderson Cancer Center
Houston, Texas
800.392.1611
mdanderson.org

University of Wisconsin
Carbone Cancer Center
Madison, Wisconsin
608.265.1700
uwhealth.org/cancer

Vanderbilt-Ingram Cancer Center
Nashville, Tennessee
800.811.8480
vicc.org

Yale Cancer Center/
Smilow Cancer Hospital
New Haven, Connecticut
855.4.SMILOW
yalecancercenter.org

Index

Made in the
USA
Columbia, SC

82347215R00027